HEALTHY MEAL FOR PREGNANT MOM

A NUTRITION GUIDE RECIPES

ANGELA HARLAN

TABLE OF CONTENTS

FRUITS

Fruits are an essential component of a healthy diet, providing a rich array of vitamins, minerals, fiber, and antioxidants. Incorporating a variety of fruits into your daily nutrition not only enhances the overall taste of your meals but also contributes to your well-being. In this exploration, we will delve into the nutritional benefits of fruits, their impact on health, and the diverse array of fruits available to us.

First and foremost, fruits are a powerhouse of vitamins. Different fruits boast various vitamins such as vitamin C, which is abundant in citrus fruits like oranges and strawberries. This vitamin is well-known for its immune-boosting properties, aiding in the body's defense against infections and promoting overall health. Additionally, fruits like bananas and avocados are rich in vitamin B6, crucial for brain development and function.

Minerals are another vital aspect of fruit nutrition. Potassium, found in fruits like bananas, helps regulate blood pressure and supports proper muscle and nerve function. Mangos and apricots, on the other hand, are excellent sources of vitamin A, contributing to healthy vision and skin. The combination of these vitamins and minerals in various fruits makes them a nutritious and well-rounded choice for a balanced diet.

Moreover, fruits are packed with dietary fiber, playing a key role in digestive health. Fiber promotes regular bowel movements, prevents constipation, and supports a healthy gut microbiome. Berries, apples, and pears are particularly high in fiber, making them valuable additions to a diet focused on digestive wellness. Including a variety of fruits can help individuals meet their daily fiber requirements, contributing to long-term gastrointestinal health.

Antioxidants are compounds found in fruits that help combat oxidative stress in the body. Oxidative stress arises from an imbalance between free radicals and antioxidants, potentially leading to various chronic diseases. Berries, such as blueberries and raspberries, are renowned for their antioxidant content, which may contribute to reducing inflammation and lowering the risk of certain illnesses. The colorful array of fruits is a testament to the diverse range of antioxidants they contain.

Beyond the nutritional benefits, fruits have been associated with numerous health advantages. Regular fruit consumption has been linked to a lower risk of heart disease, stroke, and certain types of cancer. The phytochemicals and bioactive compounds in fruits contribute to these protective effects, emphasizing the importance of including a variety of fruits in one's diet for overall well-being.

It's worth noting that while fresh fruits are often the go-to choice, frozen and dried fruits also offer nutritional benefits. Frozen fruits retain their nutrient content and can be a convenient option, especially when certain fruits are out of season. Dried fruits, though higher in sugar concentration, provide a concentrated source of vitamins and minerals.

When considering the variety of fruits available, the choices are vast and diverse. Citrus fruits like oranges, grapefruits, and lemons are not only refreshing but also high in vitamin C. Berries, including strawberries, blueberries, and raspberries, are not only delicious but also rich in antioxidants. Tropical fruits such as pineapples, mangos, and papayas bring a burst of flavor and provide unique nutrients like vitamin A and vitamin C.

Apples and pears, with their high fiber content, make for satisfying snacks that contribute to digestive health. Bananas, known for their potassium content, offer a quick and portable energy boost. Avocados, often mistaken for vegetables, are nutrient-dense fruits containing healthy monounsaturated fats, contributing to heart health and satiety.

 fruits are a treasure trove of essential nutrients that contribute to overall health and well-being. From vitamins and minerals to fiber and antioxidants, the nutritional benefits of incorporating a diverse array of fruits into your diet are abundant. Whether enjoyed fresh, frozen, or dried, the versatility of fruits makes them a delicious and accessible choice for individuals seeking a nutrient-rich and health-promoting diet. So, go ahead, embrace the vibrant spectrum of fruits available, and relish the numerous flavors and health benefits they bring to your table.

VEGETABLES

Vegetables, often referred to as nature's nutritional powerhouses, play a fundamental role in promoting overall health and well-being. Packed with essential vitamins, minerals, fiber, and antioxidants, vegetables offer a diverse array of flavors, textures, and colors that make them a cornerstone of a balanced and nutritious diet. In this exploration, we will delve into the extensive world of vegetables, examining their nutritional benefits, the impact on health, and the multitude of vegetables available to us.

One of the key attributes of vegetables is their rich vitamin content. These essential nutrients contribute to various physiological functions in the body. For instance, leafy greens like spinach and kale are abundant in vitamin K, vital for blood clotting and bone health. Bell peppers and broccoli are excellent sources of vitamin C, an antioxidant that supports the immune system, skin health, and overall well-being.

Minerals are another essential component of vegetables. Potassium, found in vegetables like sweet potatoes and tomatoes, is crucial for maintaining healthy blood pressure and supporting proper muscle and nerve function. Leafy greens such as Swiss chard and collard greens provide an abundance of calcium, contributing to bone health and muscle function.

Fiber, a non-digestible carbohydrate present in vegetables, is integral to digestive health. Vegetables like carrots, celery, and Brussels sprouts are rich in fiber, promoting regular bowel movements, preventing constipation, and supporting a healthy gut microbiome. Including a variety of vegetables in one's diet ensures an adequate intake of fiber, which is essential for overall gastrointestinal well-being.

Antioxidants, compounds that help neutralize harmful free radicals in the body, are prevalent in vegetables. Tomatoes, for example, contain the antioxidant lycopene, which has been linked to a reduced risk of certain cancers. Cruciferous vegetables like broccoli and cauliflower boast sulfur-containing compounds that may have protective effects against chronic diseases. The colorful palette of vegetables reflects the diverse range of antioxidants they offer.

Moreover, vegetables contribute to hydration as many of them have high water content. Cucumbers, zucchini, and lettuce are examples of vegetables that can contribute to daily fluid intake, supporting overall hydration and aiding in various bodily functions.

The health benefits of vegetables extend beyond their nutritional profile. Regular consumption of vegetables has been associated with a lower risk of chronic diseases, including cardiovascular diseases and certain types of cancer. The dietary fiber, vitamins, and antioxidants in vegetables collectively contribute to these protective effects, emphasizing the importance of incorporating a variety of vegetables into one's daily meals.

When exploring the vast world of vegetables, the choices are diverse, ranging from leafy greens to root vegetables. Leafy greens such as spinach, kale, and Swiss chard are nutrient-dense options, providing an array of vitamins and minerals. Root vegetables like carrots, sweet potatoes, and beets offer a natural sweetness along with essential nutrients like beta-carotene and potassium.

Cruciferous vegetables, including broccoli, cauliflower, and Brussels sprouts, are known for their unique flavors and potential health benefits. These vegetables contain compounds like glucosinolates, which may have anti-cancer properties. Allium vegetables, such as garlic, onions, and leeks, contribute not only to flavor but also provide sulfur-containing compounds with potential health-promoting effects.

Additionally, peppers—whether bell peppers, chili peppers, or sweet peppers—add vibrancy to dishes and supply a wealth of vitamins and antioxidants. Tomatoes, technically a fruit but often treated as a vegetable, are versatile and rich in lycopene. Eggplants, known for their deep purple color, offer dietary fiber and various vitamins.

The cooking methods employed can also influence the nutritional composition of vegetables. While some nutrients may be lost during cooking, certain cooking methods can enhance the bioavailability of others. For instance, lightly steaming vegetables helps retain more nutrients compared to boiling, and roasting can enhance the flavor and texture of vegetables while preserving their nutritional content.

vegetables stand as a crucial pillar of a nutritious diet, offering a plethora of vitamins, minerals, fiber, and antioxidants. From leafy greens to root vegetables, the diverse array of options allows individuals to create meals that are both delicious and nutritionally rich.

Regular consumption of vegetables not only contributes to physical health but also adds variety and color to meals, making the overall dining experience more enjoyable. So, embrace the abundance of vegetables available, experiment with different varieties, and savor the multitude of flavors and health benefits they bring to your table.

WHOLE GRAINS

Whole grains represent a fundamental category of foods that contribute significantly to a balanced and nutritious diet. Consisting of grains that retain their bran, germ, and endosperm, whole grains are rich in essential nutrients, dietary fiber, and various bioactive compounds. In this exploration, we will delve into the extensive world of whole grains, examining their nutritional benefits, impact on health, and the diverse range of options available to individuals seeking to enhance their well-being through dietary choices.

Whole grains serve as a vital source of complex carbohydrates, supplying the body with a steady release of energy. Unlike refined grains, which have had their bran and germ removed during processing, whole grains maintain these nutrient-rich components, providing a more comprehensive nutritional profile. Common whole grains include brown rice, quinoa, oats, barley, and whole wheat.

One of the primary nutritional benefits of whole grains lies in their fiber content. Dietary fiber, found in the bran and outer layer of whole grains, plays a crucial role in digestive health. It promotes regular bowel movements, helps prevent constipation, and supports a healthy gut microbiome. Consuming an adequate amount of fiber from whole grains is associated with a reduced risk of developing various gastrointestinal issues and contributes to overall digestive well-being.

Whole grains are also rich in essential vitamins and minerals. B vitamins, such as B1 (thiamine), B2 (riboflavin), B3 (niacin), and B6 (pyridoxine), are abundant in whole grains and are essential for energy metabolism, nervous system function, and the formation of red blood cells. Minerals like iron, magnesium, and zinc are also present in whole grains, contributing to various physiological processes, including oxygen transport, bone health, and immune function.

The presence of antioxidants in whole grains further enhances their nutritional value. Antioxidants help neutralize harmful free radicals in the body, reducing oxidative stress and lowering the risk of chronic diseases. For example, the outer layer of whole grains contains phenolic compounds, which have been associated with potential health benefits, including anti-inflammatory and anti-cancer properties.

Whole grains have been linked to numerous health benefits, particularly in the context of chronic disease prevention. Regular consumption of whole grains is associated with a reduced risk of heart disease, type 2 diabetes, and certain types of cancer. The combination of fiber, vitamins, minerals, and antioxidants in whole grains contributes to these protective effects, highlighting their importance in promoting long-term health.

When exploring the diverse world of whole grains, the options are extensive and varied. Brown rice, a staple in many cuisines, is a whole grain rich in fiber and provides a nutty flavor. Quinoa, considered a complete protein source, is gluten-free and contains all nine essential amino acids. Oats, whether in the form of rolled oats or steel-cut oats, are versatile and can be used in various dishes, contributing to heart health due to their beta-glucan content.

Barley, with its chewy texture, is not only rich in fiber but also contains beta-glucans and antioxidants. Whole wheat, commonly used in bread and pasta, retains the bran and germ, providing a more nutrient-dense option compared to refined wheat products. Farro, an ancient grain, adds a nutty flavor to dishes and is a good source of fiber, protein, and various nutrients.

The preparation methods of whole grains also influence their nutritional impact. Cooking methods such as boiling, steaming, or baking can help preserve the nutrient content of whole grains. However, soaking or fermenting grains before cooking can enhance nutrient bioavailability by reducing anti-nutrients, compounds that can hinder the absorption of certain nutrients.

Whole grains can be incorporated into various meals, from breakfast to dinner. Breakfast options may include oatmeal, whole grain cereal, or whole grain toast. Lunch and dinner can feature dishes with quinoa, brown rice, or whole wheat pasta. Snacks can involve whole grain crackers or popcorn. The versatility of whole grains allows for creativity in the kitchen while ensuring a diverse and nutrient-rich diet.

whole grains stand as a cornerstone of a healthful diet, offering a plethora of essential nutrients, dietary fiber, and antioxidants. From brown rice to quinoa, the diverse array of whole grains allows individuals to tailor their choices to personal preferences and dietary needs.

Regular consumption of whole grains contributes to digestive health, provides sustained energy, and offers protection against chronic diseases. Embracing the wealth of whole grains available and incorporating them into daily meals can significantly enhance overall well-being, making them an integral component of a nutritious and balanced diet.

PROTEIN

Protein, an essential macronutrient, is a crucial building block for the human body, contributing to various physiological functions, growth, and overall health. Comprising amino acids, proteins play a pivotal role in the formation of tissues, enzymes, hormones, and immune system components. In this comprehensive exploration, we will delve into the intricate world of protein, examining its diverse sources, nutritional significance, impact on health, and the importance of adequate protein intake in maintaining a balanced and thriving lifestyle.

Structure and Function of Proteins:
Proteins are composed of amino acids, which are organic compounds containing carbon, hydrogen, oxygen, nitrogen, and occasionally sulfur. These amino acids serve as the building blocks of proteins, and their unique sequences determine the structure and function of each protein in the body. There are twenty different amino acids, and the human body can produce some of them, known as non-essential amino acids. However, essential amino acids, which the body cannot produce, must be obtained through the diet.
The three-dimensional structure of proteins is critical to their function. Proteins can be globular or fibrous, and this structure is intricately related to their specific roles in the body. Enzymes, for example, are proteins that catalyze biochemical reactions, while antibodies play a

key role in the immune system's defense against pathogens.

Diverse Sources of Protein:
Proteins are abundant in a wide range of food sources, both animal and plant-based. Animal sources include meat, poultry, fish, eggs, and dairy products. These foods are considered complete proteins as they contain all essential amino acids in sufficient amounts. On the other hand, plant-based sources like legumes, nuts, seeds, grains, and vegetables also contribute valuable protein but may lack some essential amino acids. Combining various plant-based protein sources can help achieve a more balanced amino acid profile.

Nutritional Significance of Protein:

Muscle Building and Repair:
Protein is crucial for muscle building and repair. When individuals engage in physical activities, especially resistance training, small amounts of muscle tissue are damaged. Protein aids in repairing and rebuilding this tissue, contributing to muscle growth and strength. Athletes, fitness enthusiasts, and individuals recovering from injuries often have increased protein requirements.

Cellular Structure and Function:
Proteins are integral to the structure and function of cells. Cell membranes, organelles, and various cellular components are composed of proteins. Additionally,

proteins serve as transporters, facilitating the movement of molecules across cell membranes.

Enzymatic Activity:
Enzymes, which are proteins, act as catalysts for biochemical reactions. They facilitate and accelerate these reactions, playing a vital role in metabolism and other physiological processes. Without enzymes, many essential functions within the body would occur too slowly to sustain life.

Hormone Production:
Several hormones, including insulin, growth hormone, and thyroid hormones, are proteins. These hormones regulate various bodily functions, such as metabolism, growth, and energy balance. Maintaining adequate protein intake supports the synthesis of these crucial signaling molecules.

Immune Function:
Antibodies, which are specialized proteins, play a central role in the immune system. They recognize and neutralize foreign invaders such as bacteria and viruses, contributing to the body's defense against infections and diseases.

Impact on Health:

Weight Management:
Protein plays a key role in weight management. It promotes satiety, reducing feelings of hunger and aiding

in weight control. Including protein-rich foods in meals and snacks can contribute to a more satisfying and balanced diet, potentially assisting those aiming for weight loss or maintenance.

Blood Sugar Regulation:
Protein can help stabilize blood sugar levels. When consumed with carbohydrates, protein slows down the absorption of glucose, preventing rapid spikes and crashes in blood sugar. This can be particularly beneficial for individuals with insulin resistance or diabetes.

Bone Health:
Protein is essential for maintaining bone health. It contributes to the formation and maintenance of bone tissue, and adequate protein intake is associated with improved bone mineral density. This is crucial for preventing conditions like osteoporosis.

Heart Health:
Including lean protein sources in the diet can positively impact heart health. Plant-based proteins, such as those from legumes and nuts, have been associated with lower cardiovascular risk. Additionally, choosing lean cuts of meat and incorporating fish into the diet can contribute to heart health.

Aging and Muscle Mass:
Protein becomes increasingly important as individuals age. Aging is often accompanied by a natural decline in

muscle mass and function, known as sarcopenia. Consuming adequate protein, especially in combination with resistance training, can help mitigate this decline and support healthy aging.

Adequate Protein Intake:
The Recommended Dietary Allowance (RDA) for protein varies based on factors such as age, sex, activity level, and overall health. Generally, adults are advised to consume 0.8 grams of protein per kilogram of body weight per day. However, individuals engaged in intense physical activity, those aiming for muscle growth, and certain populations such as pregnant women may require higher protein intake.
It's important to distribute protein intake throughout the day to optimize its utilization by the body. Including protein-rich foods in each meal and snack helps maintain a consistent supply of amino acids for various physiological functions.

Animal-Based Protein Sources:

Meat:
Meat is a rich source of high-quality protein, as well as essential nutrients such as iron, zinc, and B vitamins. Lean cuts of meat, such as chicken breast or turkey, provide protein with lower saturated fat content.

Poultry:
Poultry, including chicken and turkey, is a popular and versatile protein source. Removing the skin and

choosing lean cuts helps minimize saturated fat intake while maximizing protein content.

Fish and Seafood:
Fish and seafood are excellent sources of protein, omega-3 fatty acids, and various minerals. Fatty fish like salmon, mackerel, and trout provide additional heart-healthy benefits.

Eggs:
Eggs are a complete protein source and also contain essential vitamins and minerals. They are versatile and can be prepared in various ways.

Dairy Products:
Dairy products, including milk, yogurt, and cheese, are rich in protein and provide calcium for bone health. Opting for low-fat or fat-free varieties helps manage overall fat intake.

Plant-Based Protein Sources:

Legumes:
Legumes, such as beans, lentils, and chickpeas, are excellent plant-based protein sources. They also offer fiber, vitamins, and minerals. Combining different legumes with grains enhances the amino acid profile.

Nuts and Seeds:

Nuts and seeds provide protein, healthy fats, and essential micronutrients. Almonds, peanuts, chia seeds, and flaxseeds are examples of nutrient-dense options.

Tofu and Tempeh:
Tofu and tempeh are soy-based products that serve as valuable protein sources for vegetarians and vegans. They are versatile ingredients in various dishes.

Quinoa:
Quinoa is a unique plant-based protein source that contains all essential amino acids, making it a complete protein. It is also rich in fiber and various minerals.

DAIRY

Dairy products play a significant role in the diets of people around the world, providing a rich source of essential nutrients, including calcium, protein, vitamins, and minerals. Derived from the milk of mammals such as cows, goats, and sheep, dairy encompasses a wide range of products consumed globally. In this comprehensive exploration, we will delve into the diverse world of dairy, examining its nutritional composition, health benefits, potential concerns, and the variety of dairy products available to consumers.

Nutritional Composition of Dairy:
Dairy products are prized for their nutrient density, offering a well-rounded package of essential nutrients crucial for overall health. The primary components of dairy include:

Calcium:
Dairy is renowned for its calcium content, a mineral vital for bone health, blood clotting, and nerve function. Adequate calcium intake is especially important during childhood and adolescence, as well as in older adults to prevent conditions like osteoporosis.

Protein:
Dairy products are excellent sources of high-quality protein, containing all essential amino acids needed for various bodily functions. Protein is essential for muscle

repair and growth, immune function, and the synthesis
of enzymes and hormones.

Vitamins:
Dairy products contain various vitamins, including B
vitamins (such as B12, riboflavin, and niacin), which
play roles in energy metabolism and the functioning of
the nervous system. Vitamin D, critical for bone health
and immune function, is often fortified in many dairy
products.

Minerals:
Besides calcium, dairy provides other minerals like
phosphorus, potassium, and magnesium. These
minerals contribute to bone health, fluid balance, and
overall metabolic functions.

Fats:
Dairy products can contain varying amounts of fats,
including saturated fats. The fat content depends on
factors like the type of milk used (whole, reduced-fat, or
skim), the processing method, and the specific dairy
product.

Common Dairy Products:

Milk:
Milk is a staple dairy product, available in various forms
such as whole milk, 2% milk, and skim milk. It serves as
a versatile ingredient, a beverage on its own, and a base
for other dairy products.

Cheese:
Cheese comes in numerous varieties, each with its unique flavor, texture, and nutritional profile. Examples include cheddar, mozzarella, feta, and Swiss. Cheese provides protein, calcium, and healthy fats.

Yogurt:
Yogurt is fermented milk that contains beneficial probiotics, which support gut health. It is a versatile dairy product that can be enjoyed on its own, as a topping, or incorporated into both sweet and savory dishes.

Butter:
Butter is a dairy product made from the fat of milk. It is commonly used in cooking, baking, and as a spread. While high in saturated fats, moderation is key for those mindful of their fat intake.

Ice Cream:
Ice cream is a popular frozen dairy dessert available in a myriad of flavors. While often considered a treat, it contributes to overall dairy consumption and provides calcium and energy.

Milk Alternatives:
With the rise of plant-based diets and lactose intolerance awareness, various milk alternatives have gained popularity. These include almond milk, soy milk, coconut milk, and oat milk. While these alternatives may

not have the same nutrient profile as dairy milk, many are fortified to provide similar benefits.

Health Benefits of Dairy:

Bone Health:
The high calcium content in dairy is essential for maintaining strong and healthy bones. Adequate calcium intake during childhood and adolescence is crucial for bone development, and continued consumption throughout life helps prevent bone-related conditions such as osteoporosis.

Protein Source:
Dairy products are excellent sources of high-quality protein, containing all essential amino acids. Protein is vital for muscle repair, growth, and overall body function. Including dairy in the diet can contribute to meeting daily protein requirements.

Nutrient Absorption:
The presence of vitamin D in many dairy products enhances calcium absorption. Vitamin D is essential for bone health and plays a role in immune function. Fortified dairy products contribute to overall vitamin D intake, especially in regions with limited sunlight.

Gut Health:
Fermented dairy products like yogurt contain probiotics, beneficial bacteria that support gut health. Probiotics

contribute to a balanced gut microbiome, potentially aiding digestion and promoting overall well-being.

Weight Management:
Some studies suggest that including dairy in a balanced diet may support weight management. The combination of protein and other nutrients in dairy products can contribute to a feeling of fullness, potentially reducing overall calorie intake.

Potential Concerns and Considerations:

Lactose Intolerance:
Lactose intolerance is a common concern, affecting individuals who lack the enzyme lactase needed to digest lactose, the sugar found in milk. For those with lactose intolerance, lactose-free dairy products or dairy alternatives can be viable options.

Saturated Fats:
Some dairy products, especially full-fat varieties, can be high in saturated fats. While saturated fats are a natural component of dairy, excessive intake may contribute to elevated cholesterol levels. Choosing low-fat or fat-free options can help manage saturated fat intake.

Cholesterol Content:
Certain dairy products, particularly those high in saturated fats, may contribute to cholesterol intake. For individuals monitoring cholesterol levels, selecting low-

fat or fat-free dairy options and moderating overall fat intake is advisable.

Allergies:
Dairy allergies, often more prevalent in childhood, involve an immune response to proteins in milk. In such cases, individuals may need to avoid all forms of dairy and use alternative sources for essential nutrients.

Diversity in Dairy Choices:
Dairy consumption is culturally influenced, and the availability of dairy products varies globally. In regions where dairy is a dietary staple, it often plays a central role in culinary traditions. However, cultural preferences, dietary restrictions, and lifestyle choices have led to an increased variety of dairy alternatives and innovative dairy-based products.

Dairy Alternatives:
The rise of dairy alternatives has expanded options for individuals with lactose intolerance, dairy allergies, or those following plant-based diets. Common dairy alternatives include:

Almond Milk:
Made from almonds, almond milk has a nutty flavor and is often fortified with calcium and vitamin D.

Soy Milk:

A protein-rich alternative made from soybeans, soy milk is a suitable replacement for cow's milk and is often fortified with essential nutrients.

Coconut Milk:
Derived from coconuts, coconut milk has a distinct tropical flavor. It is commonly used in both sweet and savory dishes.

Oat Milk:
Made from oats, oat milk has gained popularity for its creamy texture. It is often fortified with vitamins and minerals.

Rice Milk:
Produced from rice, rice milk is a dairy-free alternative. It tends to be thinner than cow's milk and is often fortified with nutrients.

Dairy products stand as a versatile and nutrient-dense category within the realm of nutrition. Whether consumed for their high calcium content, protein richness, or cultural significance, dairy plays a vital role in supporting overall health.

LEGUMES

Legumes, a diverse group of plant species that bear fruit in the form of pods, are an integral component of diets worldwide. These nutritionally dense seeds, commonly known as pulses, encompass a wide variety of beans, lentils, peas, and chickpeas. In this comprehensive exploration, we will delve into the extensive world of legumes, examining their nutritional profile, health benefits, culinary versatility, and their impact on sustainable agriculture.

Nutritional Profile:
Legumes are renowned for their impressive nutritional composition, making them an excellent source of essential nutrients. Some key components include:

Protein:
Legumes are rich in plant-based protein, making them an essential dietary component for vegetarians and vegans. They provide a valuable protein source with amino acids crucial for various physiological functions, including muscle development and repair.

Dietary Fiber:
Legumes are high in dietary fiber, both soluble and insoluble. Fiber promotes digestive health, helps regulate blood sugar levels, and contributes to a feeling of fullness, making legumes an excellent choice for weight management.

Complex Carbohydrates:
Legumes offer complex carbohydrates, providing a sustained release of energy. This makes them an ideal choice for individuals seeking stable blood sugar levels and prolonged satiety.

Micronutrients:
Legumes contain essential micronutrients such as folate, iron, magnesium, potassium, and zinc. These nutrients contribute to various bodily functions, including red blood cell formation, immune support, and bone health.

Antioxidants:
Legumes contain a variety of antioxidants, including flavonoids and polyphenols. These compounds help neutralize free radicals in the body, potentially reducing the risk of chronic diseases.

Common Types of Legumes:

Beans:
Black Beans: Rich in protein, fiber, and antioxidants, black beans are a versatile legume used in a variety of dishes.
Kidney Beans: Kidney beans are known for their kidney-like shape and provide a good source of plant-based protein.
Chickpeas: Chickpeas, or garbanzo beans, are versatile and commonly used in salads, stews, and as the main ingredient in hummus.

Lentils: Lentils come in various colors and are a quick-cooking source of protein, fiber, and essential nutrients.

Peas:
Green Peas: These sweet and vibrant peas are commonly used in a variety of dishes, from side dishes to soups and salads.
Split Peas: Split peas are hulled and split, often used in soups and stews, providing a good source of protein and fiber.

Soybeans:
Edamame: Young, green soybeans are a popular snack and appetizer. They are rich in protein and can be enjoyed boiled or steamed.
Tofu: Tofu, made from soybean curds, is a versatile and protein-rich ingredient used in various cuisines.

Lupins:
Lupini Beans: Commonly consumed in Mediterranean and Middle Eastern cuisines, lupini beans are known for their high protein and fiber content.

Peanuts:
Peanuts: Although technically a legume, peanuts are often categorized with nuts. They are rich in protein, healthy fats, and various essential nutrients.

Health Benefits:

Heart Health:

Legumes contribute to heart health by promoting healthy cholesterol levels. The soluble fiber they contain helps lower LDL cholesterol, reducing the risk of cardiovascular diseases.

Weight Management:
The combination of protein and fiber in legumes makes them particularly satiating, aiding in weight management by promoting a feeling of fullness and reducing overall calorie intake.

Blood Sugar Regulation:
The complex carbohydrates and fiber in legumes contribute to stable blood sugar levels. This can be beneficial for individuals with diabetes or those aiming to prevent insulin resistance.

Digestive Health:
Legumes, rich in dietary fiber, support digestive health by preventing constipation and promoting regular bowel movements. Fiber also nourishes beneficial gut bacteria.

Reduced Risk of Chronic Diseases:
The antioxidants present in legumes contribute to reducing oxidative stress, potentially lowering the risk of chronic diseases such as certain cancers and inflammatory conditions.

Culinary Versatility:
Legumes boast remarkable culinary versatility, featuring prominently in various traditional dishes worldwide.

Their adaptability makes them suitable for a wide range of cuisines and cooking methods. Some popular ways to incorporate legumes into meals include:

Soups and Stews:
Legumes add heartiness and nutritional value to soups and stews. Dishes like lentil soup, split pea soup, and chili are classic examples.

Salads:
Legumes, particularly chickpeas, lentils, and beans, enhance the protein and fiber content of salads. They add texture and make salads more satisfying.

Curries and Stir-Fries:
Legumes contribute to the protein content of curries and stir-fries. Chickpeas, lentils, and tofu are popular choices for these flavorful dishes.

Dips and Spreads:
Hummus, a spread made from chickpeas, is a widely enjoyed dip. Similarly, black bean dip and lentil hummus showcase the versatility of legumes in creating delicious spreads.

Burgers and Patties:
Legumes, especially black beans and lentils, can be used to create vegetarian burgers and patties. These alternatives provide a protein-packed and plant-based option.

Baked Goods:
Incorporating legume flours, such as chickpea flour or lentil flour, into baking recipes adds a nutritional boost. This is a gluten-free option that enhances the protein and fiber content of baked goods.

Sustainable Agriculture:
Beyond their nutritional benefits, legumes play a crucial role in sustainable agriculture. They contribute to soil health and fertility through a process known as nitrogen fixation. Legumes form a symbiotic relationship with nitrogen-fixing bacteria, allowing them to convert atmospheric nitrogen into a form usable by plants. This process enhances soil fertility, reducing the need for synthetic fertilizers and promoting sustainable farming practices.

Legumes, with their exceptional nutritional profile, health benefits, and culinary versatility, stand as a cornerstone of balanced and sustainable diets. Whether enjoyed in traditional dishes, innovative recipes, or plant-based alternatives, legumes offer a wealth of nutrients, including protein, fiber, vitamins, and minerals. Incorporating a variety of legumes into daily meals not only contributes to individual well-being but also supports sustainable agricultural practices, making them a valuable and accessible food source for diverse populations worldwide.

NUTS AND SEEDS

Nuts and seeds are nutritional powerhouses, packed with a diverse array of essential nutrients that contribute to overall health and well-being. These small but mighty plant-based foods come in various shapes, sizes, and flavors, providing a rich source of healthy fats, protein, vitamins, minerals, and antioxidants. In this comprehensive exploration, we will delve into the extensive world of nuts and seeds, examining their nutritional benefits, potential health effects, culinary versatility, and their role in promoting a balanced and nutritious diet.

Nutritional Composition:
Nuts:

Almonds:
Almonds are rich in monounsaturated fats, vitamin E, magnesium, and fiber.
They provide a good source of protein and are associated with heart health benefits.

Walnuts:
Walnuts are high in omega-3 fatty acids, particularly alpha-linolenic acid (ALA).
They also contain antioxidants, vitamin E, and manganese.

Cashews:

Cashews are a good source of monounsaturated fats and copper.
They provide iron, zinc, and magnesium, contributing to immune function and overall health.

Pistachios:
Pistachios contain healthy fats, protein, and dietary fiber.
They provide essential nutrients, including vitamin B6, copper, and manganese.

Brazil Nuts:
Brazil nuts are known for their high selenium content, a mineral crucial for antioxidant defense and thyroid function.
They also provide healthy fats, protein, and essential minerals.

Seeds:

Chia Seeds:
Chia seeds are rich in omega-3 fatty acids, fiber, and protein.
They absorb liquid, forming a gel-like consistency, making them versatile for various recipes.

Flaxseeds:
Flaxseeds are a rich source of alpha-linolenic acid (ALA), lignans, and fiber.
They have been associated with heart health benefits and may have anti-inflammatory effects.

Sunflower Seeds:
Sunflower seeds are high in vitamin E, copper, and selenium.
They provide healthy fats, protein, and are a good source of antioxidants.

Pumpkin Seeds (Pepitas):
Pumpkin seeds are rich in magnesium, zinc, and iron.
They also provide protein, healthy fats, and antioxidants.

Sesame Seeds:
Sesame seeds are a good source of copper, manganese, and calcium.
They contain lignans, which may have antioxidant and anti-inflammatory properties.

Health Benefits:

Heart Health:

Omega-3 Fatty Acids:
Nuts and seeds, especially walnuts, chia seeds, and flaxseeds, are rich sources of omega-3 fatty acids. These fats have been associated with cardiovascular health, reducing the risk of heart disease.

Monounsaturated Fats:

Many nuts, such as almonds and cashews, contain monounsaturated fats. These fats are heart-healthy and may contribute to improved lipid profiles.

Weight Management:

Satiety and Fullness:
The combination of healthy fats, protein, and fiber in nuts and seeds contributes to a feeling of fullness, potentially reducing overall calorie intake. This can be beneficial for weight management.

Metabolic Rate:
Some studies suggest that the inclusion of nuts in the diet may not lead to weight gain and may even enhance metabolic rate, supporting weight maintenance.

Blood Sugar Regulation:

Fiber Content:
The fiber in nuts and seeds, such as chia seeds and flaxseeds, aids in regulating blood sugar levels. Fiber slows down the absorption of glucose, contributing to stable blood sugar.

Magnesium:
Nuts and seeds, including almonds and pumpkin seeds, are good sources of magnesium. Magnesium plays a role in insulin sensitivity, contributing to blood sugar regulation.

Anti-Inflammatory Effects:

Omega-3 Fatty Acids:
The omega-3 fatty acids in certain nuts and seeds, particularly walnuts and flaxseeds, may have anti-inflammatory effects, potentially reducing the risk of chronic diseases.

Antioxidants:
Nuts and seeds contain antioxidants, such as vitamin E and selenium, which contribute to reducing oxidative stress and inflammation in the body.

Bone Health:

Calcium and Magnesium:

Sesame seeds are rich in calcium, contributing to bone health. Additionally, magnesium in nuts and seeds supports calcium absorption and bone mineralization.

Phosphorus:
Pumpkin seeds provide phosphorus, another essential mineral for bone health and structure.

Culinary Versatility:
Nuts and seeds offer endless possibilities in the kitchen, enhancing both sweet and savory dishes. Their versatility allows for creative culinary exploration, and they can be enjoyed in various forms:

Snacking:
Nuts and seeds make for convenient and nutritious snacks. Whether eaten raw, roasted, or flavored, they provide a satisfying crunch and a nutrient boost.

Trail Mixes:
Creating personalized trail mixes with a combination of nuts, seeds, and dried fruits allows for a customizable and energy-boosting snack.

Smoothie Additions:
Adding chia seeds, flaxseeds, or nut butters to smoothies increases their nutritional content, providing healthy fats, protein, and added texture.

Salads:
Nuts and seeds, when toasted or roasted, add a delightful crunch to salads. They also contribute to the overall flavor profile.

Baking:
Incorporating nuts and seeds into baked goods, such as muffins, granola bars, and bread, not only enhances taste but also provides additional nutrients.

Nut and Seed Butters:
Nut butters, including almond butter, peanut butter, and sunflower seed butter, are versatile spreads that can be used in sandwiches, as dips, or as ingredients in various recipes.

Concerns and Considerations:

Caloric Density:
While nuts and seeds are nutrient-dense, they are also calorie-dense. Portion control is important, especially for individuals watching their calorie intake.

Allergies:
Some individuals may have allergies to certain nuts or seeds. It's crucial to be aware of allergies and choose alternatives accordingly.

Added Ingredients:
Some commercially available nuts and seeds may have added ingredients such as salt, sugar, or oil. Opting for unsalted and minimally processed varieties is recommended.

Nuts and seeds, with their nutritional richness and versatility, are invaluable additions to a balanced and healthful diet. From heart-healthy fats to protein, fiber, and an array of essential nutrients, these plant-based foods offer a multitude of health benefits. Whether enjoyed as a snack, incorporated into meals, or used in baking, nuts and seeds contribute to both the culinary experience and overall well-being.

HEALTHY FATS

Healthy fats play a crucial role in maintaining overall health and well-being. These fats, also known as unsaturated fats, come in various forms and are essential for several physiological functions within the body. In this comprehensive exploration, we will delve into the extensive world of healthy fats, examining their classification, nutritional significance, sources, and the impact of incorporating them into a balanced and nutritious diet.

Classification of Fats:

Saturated Fats:
Saturated fats are typically solid at room temperature and are commonly found in animal-based products such as meat, dairy, and certain tropical oils like coconut oil and palm oil. While small amounts of saturated fats are necessary for specific bodily functions, excessive intake has been associated with an increased risk of cardiovascular diseases.

 Unsaturated Fats:
Unsaturated fats include both monounsaturated fats and polyunsaturated fats. These fats are typically liquid at room temperature and are considered heart-healthy when consumed in moderation.

Monounsaturated Fats:

Monounsaturated fats are found in various plant-based oils, nuts, seeds, and certain fruits like avocados. These fats have been linked to improved heart health and may help lower LDL (low-density lipoprotein) cholesterol levels.

Polyunsaturated Fats:
Polyunsaturated fats include omega-3 and omega-6 fatty acids. Sources of omega-3 fatty acids include fatty fish (such as salmon and mackerel), flaxseeds, chia seeds, and walnuts. Omega-6 fatty acids are present in vegetable oils, nuts, and seeds. Both omega-3 and omega-6 fatty acids play vital roles in supporting brain function, reducing inflammation, and maintaining cardiovascular health.

Nutritional Significance:

Energy Source:
Fats are a concentrated source of energy, providing more than twice the calories per gram compared to carbohydrates and proteins. They serve as a long-lasting and efficient fuel reserve for the body.

Cell Structure:
Healthy fats are integral to the structure of cell membranes. They contribute to the flexibility and functionality of cell membranes, facilitating various cellular processes and ensuring proper communication between cells.

Nutrient Absorption:
Fats play a crucial role in the absorption of fat-soluble vitamins—vitamins A, D, E, and K. These vitamins are essential for various bodily functions, including vision, bone health, antioxidant defense, and blood clotting.

Hormone Production:
Fats are involved in the synthesis of hormones, including steroid hormones such as estrogen and testosterone. Hormones play key roles in regulating metabolism, reproductive processes, and overall physiological balance.

Brain Function:
The brain is composed of a significant amount of fat, and maintaining an adequate intake of healthy fats is essential for cognitive function and overall brain health. Omega-3 fatty acids, in particular, are crucial for brain development and function.

Heart Health:
Consuming healthy fats, particularly monounsaturated and polyunsaturated fats, has been associated with improved heart health. These fats can help lower LDL cholesterol levels, reduce inflammation, and contribute to overall cardiovascular well-being.

Anti-Inflammatory Properties:
Omega-3 fatty acids, found in fatty fish, flaxseeds, and walnuts, have anti-inflammatory properties. They may help mitigate inflammation in the body, potentially

reducing the risk of chronic diseases associated with inflammation.

Sources of Healthy Fats:

Fatty Fish:
Fatty fish, such as salmon, mackerel, sardines, and trout, are rich sources of omega-3 fatty acids. Including these fish in the diet can contribute to cardiovascular health and support brain function.

Nuts and Seeds:
Almonds: Almonds are a great source of monounsaturated fats, vitamin E, and magnesium.
Walnuts: Walnuts contain omega-3 fatty acids, antioxidants, and other essential nutrients.
Chia Seeds: Chia seeds are rich in omega-3 fatty acids, fiber, and protein.
Flaxseeds: Flaxseeds provide omega-3 fatty acids, lignans, and dietary fiber.
Sunflower Seeds: Sunflower seeds offer a combination of healthy fats, vitamins, and minerals.

Avocados:
Avocados are packed with monounsaturated fats, which contribute to heart health. They also provide potassium, vitamin K, and folate.

Olive Oil:

Olive oil, especially extra virgin olive oil, is a staple in the Mediterranean diet. It is high in monounsaturated fats and antioxidants, contributing to heart health.

Coconut Oil:
While coconut oil contains saturated fats, it is unique due to its composition of medium-chain triglycerides (MCTs). Some studies suggest potential benefits, but moderation is advised due to its saturated fat content.

Nut Butters:
Nut butters, such as almond butter and peanut butter, are sources of healthy fats, protein, and essential nutrients. Choosing varieties without added sugars or hydrogenated oils is recommended.

Seeds and Legumes:
Chia Seeds: Chia seeds provide omega-3 fatty acids, fiber, and protein.
Flaxseeds: Flaxseeds offer omega-3 fatty acids, lignans, and dietary fiber.
Sesame Seeds: Sesame seeds contain monounsaturated fats, vitamins, and minerals.

Dark Chocolate:
Dark chocolate, in moderation, contains monounsaturated fats and antioxidants. Choosing chocolate with higher cocoa content provides more health benefits.

Incorporating Healthy Fats into the Diet:

Cooking Oils:
Choose healthy cooking oils such as olive oil, avocado oil, and canola oil for sautéing, baking, and dressing salads.

Fatty Fish:
Include fatty fish like salmon, mackerel, and sardines in your diet regularly. Aim for at least two servings of fatty fish per week.

Nuts and Seeds:
Snack on a handful of nuts or seeds, add them to salads, yogurt, or include them in smoothies for an extra nutritional boost.

Avocado:
Enjoy avocados as a spread on toast, sliced in salads, or as a creamy addition to various dishes.

Nut Butters:
Spread nut butters on whole-grain bread, use them as a dip for fruit or vegetables, or incorporate them into smoothies.

Olive Oil-Based Dressings:
Make salad dressings using extra virgin olive oil and balsamic vinegar for a flavorful and heart-healthy option.

Dark Chocolate:

Indulge in moderate amounts of dark chocolate with higher cocoa content as a delicious and satisfying treat.

Concerns and Considerations:
Portion Control:
While healthy fats offer numerous benefits, it's important to consume them in moderation. Being mindful of portion sizes prevents excessive calorie intake.

CALCIUM-RICH FOODS

Calcium is a vital mineral that plays a fundamental role in various physiological functions within the body, particularly in bone and teeth formation, blood clotting, muscle function, and nerve transmission. Ensuring an adequate intake of calcium is crucial for overall health and well-being. In this comprehensive exploration, we will delve into the extensive world of calcium-rich foods, examining their nutritional significance, sources, absorption factors, and the impact of incorporating them into a balanced and nutritious diet.

Nutritional Significance of Calcium:

Bone Health:
Calcium is a primary component of bones and teeth, providing structural support and strength. Adequate calcium intake during childhood and adolescence is especially critical for the development of strong and healthy bones. As individuals age, maintaining sufficient calcium levels becomes essential to prevent bone loss and conditions such as osteoporosis.

Blood Clotting:
Calcium plays a crucial role in the blood clotting process. It is involved in the activation of various clotting factors, which help control bleeding and promote wound healing.

Muscle Function:
Calcium is essential for muscle contraction and relaxation. When nerve signals stimulate muscles, calcium is released, allowing the muscle fibers to contract. The subsequent removal of calcium enables muscle relaxation.

Nerve Transmission:
Calcium ions are vital for the transmission of nerve impulses. They assist in the release of neurotransmitters, facilitating communication between nerve cells and allowing the transmission of signals throughout the nervous system.

Cellular Function:
Calcium acts as a secondary messenger in numerous cellular processes, including enzyme activation, hormone secretion, and cell signaling. Maintaining an appropriate balance of calcium within cells is crucial for their proper function.

Calcium-Rich Foods:

Dairy Products:
Milk: Milk is a rich source of calcium, providing about 300 mg per cup. It also contains vitamin D, which enhances calcium absorption.
Yogurt: Yogurt is a versatile dairy product that contains probiotics, beneficial bacteria that support gut health, along with calcium.

Cheese: Various types of cheese, such as cheddar, mozzarella, and Swiss, are good sources of calcium. However, their calcium content may vary.

 Leafy Green Vegetables:
Kale: Kale is a nutrient-dense leafy green that provides a significant amount of calcium per serving. It also offers other essential vitamins and minerals.
Collard Greens: Collard greens are rich in calcium and are a staple in many cuisines, especially in Southern cooking.
Spinach: While spinach contains calcium, it also contains oxalates that may interfere with calcium absorption. Cooking can help reduce oxalate levels.

Fish:
Salmon and Sardines: Fatty fish like salmon and sardines not only provide omega-3 fatty acids but are also excellent sources of calcium due to their edible bones.

Fortified Foods:
Fortified Plant-Based Milk: Many plant-based milk alternatives, such as almond milk, soy milk, and oat milk, are often fortified with calcium and vitamin D to provide similar nutritional benefits as dairy milk.
Fortified Cereals: Certain breakfast cereals are fortified with calcium and other nutrients. Checking food labels can help identify fortified options.

Nuts and Seeds:

Almonds: Almonds are not only a good source of healthy fats but also provide a notable amount of calcium.
Chia Seeds: Chia seeds offer a combination of calcium, omega-3 fatty acids, and dietary fiber.

Tofu and Soy Products:
Tofu: Tofu, made from soybeans, is a versatile plant-based source of calcium. It is often used in vegetarian and vegan dishes.
Edamame: Young soybeans, known as edamame, are another calcium-rich option.

Legumes:
White Beans: White beans, including navy beans and cannellini beans, are rich in calcium, making them a nutritious addition to various dishes.
Chickpeas: Chickpeas, or garbanzo beans, provide calcium along with protein and fiber.

Fortified Beverages:
Fortified Orange Juice: Some brands of orange juice are fortified with calcium and vitamin D, providing a refreshing way to supplement calcium intake.

Calcium Absorption Factors:

Vitamin D:
Vitamin D enhances calcium absorption in the intestines. Exposure to sunlight is a natural way to synthesize vitamin D, and it is also found in certain

foods, including fatty fish, egg yolks, and fortified dairy products.

Magnesium:
Magnesium plays a supportive role in calcium absorption. Including magnesium-rich foods, such as nuts, seeds, whole grains, and leafy green vegetables, can contribute to overall bone health.

Vitamin K:
Vitamin K is involved in bone metabolism and may play a role in calcium regulation. Leafy green vegetables, broccoli, and Brussels sprouts are good sources of vitamin K.

 Calcium-to-Phosphorus Ratio:
Balancing the intake of calcium with an adequate intake of phosphorus is important for optimal absorption. Dairy products, fish, and poultry provide a naturally balanced ratio.

Oxalates and Phytates:
Oxalates, found in certain vegetables like spinach, and phytates, found in whole grains and legumes, can bind to calcium and inhibit its absorption. Cooking can help reduce oxalate levels, and soaking or fermenting can decrease phytate content.

Calcium Requirements:
The Recommended Dietary Allowance (RDA) for calcium varies by age and gender. It is important to note

that individual requirements may differ based on factors such as activity level, life stage (e.g., pregnancy or lactation), and overall health.

Infants:
0 to 6 months: 200 mg
7 to 12 months: 260 mg

Children:
1 to 3 years: 700 mg
4 to 8 years: 1,000 mg
9 to 13 years: 1,300 mg

 Adolescents and Adults:
14 to 18 years: 1,300 mg
19 to 50 years: 1,000 mg (male and female)
51 to 70 years: 1,000 mg (male), 1,200 mg (female)

years and older: 1,200 mg
4. Pregnancy and Lactation:
14 to 18 years: 1,300 mg (pregnancy), 1,300 mg (lactation)
19 to 50 years: 1,000 mg (pregnancy), 1,000 mg (lactation)

Calcium-rich foods are essential components of a well-balanced diet, contributing to various physiological functions within the body.

IRON-RICH FOODS

Iron is a vital mineral that plays a crucial role in numerous physiological processes within the body, including oxygen transport, energy metabolism, and immune function. Ensuring an adequate intake of iron is essential for overall health and well-being. In this comprehensive exploration, we will delve into the extensive world of iron-rich foods, examining their nutritional significance, sources, absorption factors, and the impact of incorporating them into a balanced and nutritious diet.

Nutritional Significance of Iron:

Oxygen Transport:
Iron is a key component of hemoglobin, a protein in red blood cells responsible for transporting oxygen from the lungs to tissues and organs throughout the body. Myoglobin, another iron-containing protein, facilitates oxygen storage and release in muscle cells.

Energy Metabolism:
Iron is involved in the production of adenosine triphosphate (ATP), the primary energy currency of cells. It plays a crucial role in the electron transport chain, contributing to energy production within mitochondria.

Immune Function:

Iron is essential for the proper functioning of the immune system. It supports the proliferation and activity of immune cells, helping the body defend against infections and illnesses.

Cognitive Development:
Adequate iron levels are particularly crucial during periods of rapid growth and development, such as infancy, childhood, and adolescence. Iron is necessary for cognitive development, learning, and overall brain function.

Pregnancy:
Iron needs increase during pregnancy to support the growing fetus and the expansion of the maternal blood volume. Insufficient iron intake during pregnancy can lead to iron deficiency anemia and negatively impact both maternal and fetal health.

Types of Dietary Iron:

Heme Iron:
Heme iron is found in animal-based foods and is more efficiently absorbed by the body compared to non-heme iron. Foods rich in heme iron include:

Red Meat: Beef, lamb, and pork are excellent sources of heme iron.
Organ Meats: Liver and other organ meats contain high levels of heme iron.

Poultry: Chicken and turkey are good sources of heme iron.

Non-Heme Iron:
Non-heme iron is present in plant-based and fortified foods. While the absorption of non-heme iron is generally lower than that of heme iron, it can be enhanced by consuming it alongside vitamin C-rich foods. Foods rich in non-heme iron include:

Legumes: Lentils, chickpeas, and beans provide significant amounts of non-heme iron.
Fortified Foods: Certain cereals, bread, and plant-based milk alternatives are fortified with iron.
Leafy Green Vegetables: Spinach, kale, and Swiss chard contain non-heme iron, although they also contain compounds that may inhibit absorption.

Iron-Rich Foods:

Red Meat:
Beef: Beef is a particularly rich source of heme iron. It also provides essential nutrients such as protein, zinc, and vitamin B12.
Lamb: Lamb is another red meat that contributes to iron intake. It is often consumed in various cuisines worldwide.

Poultry:

Chicken: Chicken, especially dark meat, contains heme iron. Removing the skin reduces the fat content while maintaining iron levels.
Turkey: Similar to chicken, turkey provides heme iron and is a lean source of protein.

Fish:
Sardines: Sardines, especially when consumed with their bones, are rich in heme iron. They also offer omega-3 fatty acids and calcium.
Tuna: Tuna is a versatile fish that provides heme iron along with protein. Canned tuna is a convenient option.

Organ Meats:
Liver: Liver, particularly beef liver, is exceptionally high in heme iron. It also contains various vitamins and minerals, including vitamin A, copper, and folate.

Legumes:
Lentils: Lentils are a plant-based source of non-heme iron. They are also rich in fiber, protein, and other essential nutrients.
Chickpeas: Chickpeas, also known as garbanzo beans, contribute to iron intake and are versatile in various dishes.

Beans:
Black Beans: Black beans provide non-heme iron along with fiber, protein, and other essential nutrients.

Kidney Beans: Kidney beans are another type of beans that contributes to iron intake. They are commonly used in various cuisines.

Nuts and Seeds:
Pumpkin Seeds: Pumpkin seeds, also known as pepitas, are a plant-based source of non-heme iron. They also provide zinc and magnesium.
Sunflower Seeds: Sunflower seeds contribute to iron intake and offer a range of nutrients, including vitamin E and selenium.

Fortified Foods:
Fortified Cereals: Many breakfast cereals are fortified with iron, making them a convenient option for boosting iron intake, especially for breakfast.
Fortified Plant-Based Milk: Some plant-based milk alternatives, such as fortified almond milk and soy milk, provide non-heme iron.

Tofu and Soy Products:
Tofu: Tofu, made from soybeans, is a versatile plant-based source of non-heme iron. It is commonly used in vegetarian and vegan diets.
Edamame: Young soybeans, known as edamame, are another plant-based source of non-heme iron.

Factors Affecting Iron Absorption:

Vitamin C:

Consuming vitamin C-rich foods alongside iron-rich plant-based foods can enhance the absorption of non-heme iron. Examples include citrus fruits, strawberries, and bell peppers.

Animal-Based Sources:
Heme iron from animal-based sources is more efficiently absorbed than non-heme iron. Including both heme and non-heme iron sources in the diet can contribute to overall iron absorption.

Calcium and Tannins:
Calcium and tannins, found in certain foods and beverages, can inhibit the absorption of both heme and nonheme iron. It's advisable to avoid consuming these substances simultaneously with iron-rich meals.

Phytates and Oxalates:
Similar to calcium and tannins, phytates (found in whole grains and legumes) and oxalates (found in certain vegetables) can bind to iron and reduce its absorption. Cooking or soaking can help reduce phytate levels.